<u>Unlock the Secrets to Living Your Best Life with Diabetes: A Comprehensive Guide to Self-Care</u>

Discover the ultimate guide to mastering diabetes self-care and unlocking your optimal health! This eBook is your one-stop resource for understanding and managing diabetes, packed with expert advice, practical tips, and inspiring stories. Dive in and learn how to take control of your health and live a vibrant, fulfilling life with diabetes.

￼ Transform your life with this persuasive title, designed to captivate your audience and inspire action! ￼My wife has had type 1 diabetes for over 30 years and I have seen first hand the struggles and triumphs of everyday.

Table of Contents

Chapter 1

Introduction

Welcome to the ultimate guide for living your best life with diabetes! This eBook is designed to empower and educate you on the essential aspects of self-care, providing you with the knowledge and tools necessary to manage your diabetes effectively and thrive.

The Importance of Diabetes Self-Care

Diabetes self-care is a critical component of managing this chronic condition. By taking an active role in your health, you can reduce the risk of complications, improve your quality of life, and enhance your overall well-being. This eBook will cover various aspects of diabetes self-care, from monitoring your blood sugar levels to building a support system and cultivating healthy habits for the long term.

Understanding Diabetes and Its Impact

Diabetes is a prevalent chronic condition affecting millions of people worldwide. It occurs when your body can't produce enough insulin or effectively use the insulin it does produce, leading to high blood sugar levels. Uncontrolled diabetes can result in severe health complications, such as heart disease, nerve damage, and kidney problems. By understanding diabetes and its impact, you can take proactive steps to manage your condition and protect your health.

What to Expect in This eBook

In the following chapters, you'll discover practical strategies, expert advice, and useful links to help you navigate your diabetes journey. From diet and exercise to mental health and medication management, this eBook covers various topics to empower you to take control of your health and live your best life with diabetes.

Chapter 2

Understanding Diabetes: Types, Causes, and Symptoms

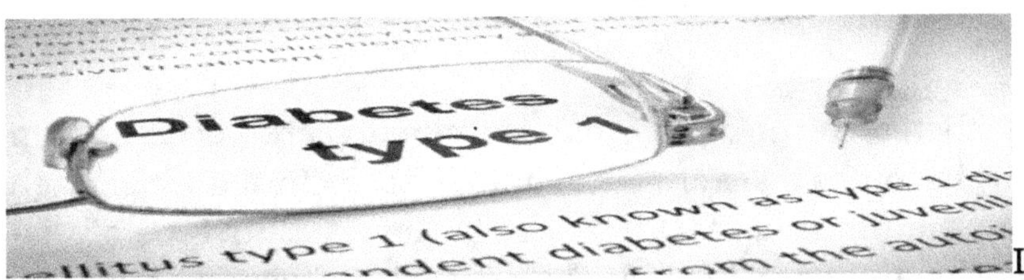

In this chapter, we will delve into the different types of diabetes, their causes, and common symptoms. By understanding these aspects, you can identify the warning signs and take appropriate action to manage your condition effectively.

Type 1 Diabetes

Type 1 diabetes, previously known as juvenile diabetes, is a condition where the pancreas produces little to no insulin. This type of diabetes typically develops in childhood or adolescence but can occur at any age. The exact cause of Type 1 diabetes is unknown, but it is believed to be caused by an autoimmune reaction that destroys the insulin-producing cells in the pancreas.

Symptoms of Type 1 Diabetes

Common symptoms of Type 1 diabetes include:

- Increased thirst and frequent urination

- Extreme hunger

- Unexplained weight loss

- Fatigue

- Irritability

- Blurred vision

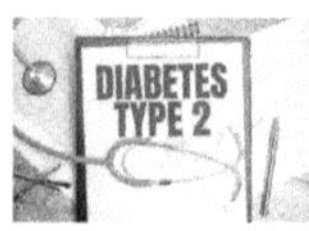

Type 2 Diabetes

Type 2 diabetes, the most common form of diabetes, occurs when your body becomes resistant to insulin or doesn't produce enough insulin to maintain normal blood sugar levels. This type of diabetes is often linked to lifestyle factors such as being overweight, inactive, or having a family history of the condition.

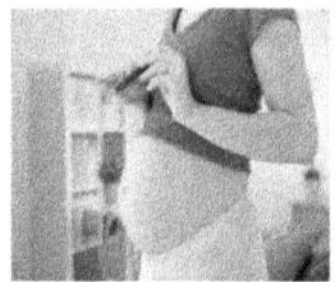

Gestational Diabetes

Gestational diabetes is a form of diabetes that develops during pregnancy. It usually goes away after the baby is born, but sometimes it doesn't and the mother develops diabetes. Women who have had gestational diabetes are at increased risk of developing Type 2 diabetes later in life.

Symptoms of Gestational Diabetes

Gestational diabetes may not cause noticeable symptoms, which is why regular screenings are essential during pregnancy. If symptoms do occur, they may include:

- Increased thirst and frequent urination
- Fatigue
- Nausea and vomiting
- Blurred vision

Pre-diabetes

Pre-diabetes is a condition where blood sugar levels are higher than normal but not high enough to be classified as diabetes. This condition often progresses to Type 2 diabetes if left untreated.

Symptoms of Pre-diabetes

Pre-diabetes typically does not cause noticeable symptoms, making regular screenings essential for early detection and prevention.

By understanding the different types of diabetes, their causes, and symptoms, you can take proactive steps to manage your condition and protect your health. In the next chapter, we will explore the importance of monitoring blood sugar, blood pressure, and other vital health indicators.

Chapter 3

The Power of Monitoring: Blood Sugar, Blood Pressure, and More

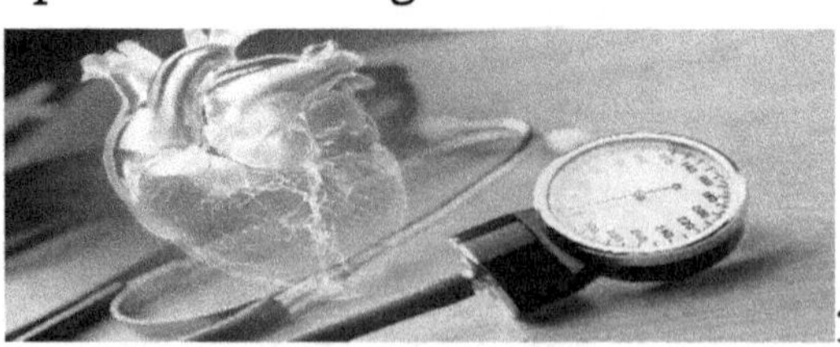In this chapter, we will discuss the importance of monitoring various health indicators, such as blood sugar, blood pressure, and cholesterol levels, to effectively manage diabetes and reduce the risk of complications.

Blood Sugar Monitoring

Regular blood sugar monitoring is crucial for managing diabetes and preventing complications. By checking your blood sugar levels frequently, you can:

1. Gain a better understanding of how different factors, such as food, exercise, and stress, affect your blood sugar levels.

2. Adjust your diet, medication, and physical activity to maintain optimal blood sugar levels.

3. Detect and treat high or low blood sugar episodes promptly.

Blood Pressure Monitoring

High blood pressure, or hypertension, is a common complication of diabetes. Regularly monitoring your blood pressure can help you:

1. Identify elevated blood pressure levels early.

2. Adjust your lifestyle and medication to lower your blood pressure and reduce the risk of complications.

Cholesterol Monitoring

People with diabetes are at an increased risk of developing high cholesterol levels, which can lead to heart disease and other complications. Regular cholesterol monitoring can help you:

1. Assess your risk of heart disease and stroke.
2. Adjust your diet, exercise, and medication to maintain healthy cholesterol levels.

Other Health Indicators

In addition to blood sugar, blood pressure, and cholesterol, other health indicators that should be monitored include:

- Kidney function: Regular testing can help detect kidney damage early and prevent further progression.

- A1C levels: This is a three-month average of your blood sugar levels, providing a broader perspective on your overall blood sugar control.

By monitoring these health indicators regularly, you can take proactive steps to manage your diabetes effectively and reduce the risk of complications. In the next chapter, we will explore the Diabetes Plate Method, a balanced and flexible approach to eating for optimal health.

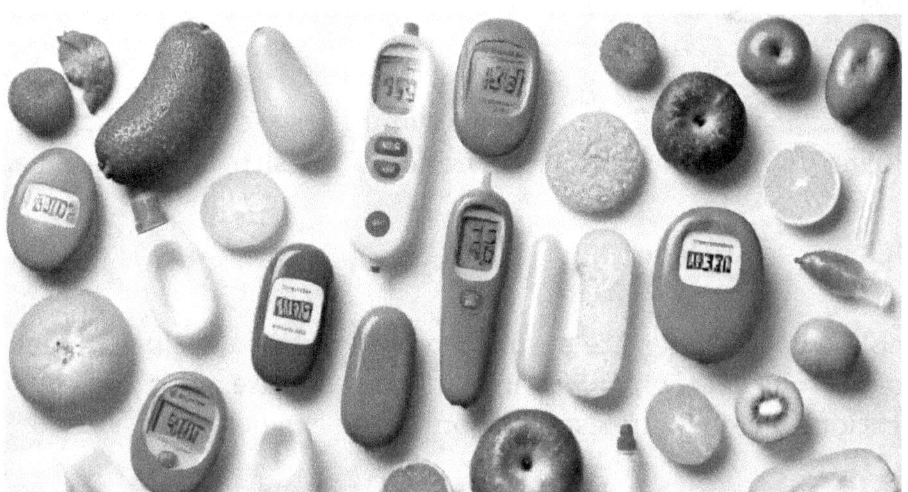

Chapter 4

The Diabetes Plate Method: Balanced Eating for Optimal Health

Eating a balanced and nutritious diet is essential for effective diabetes management. The Diabetes Plate Method is a simple and effective way to plan balanced meals that help maintain optimal blood sugar levels.

The Diabetes Plate Method involves dividing your plate into three sections:

1.   Non-starchy vegetables: Fill half of your plate with non-starchy vegetables, such as broccoli, spinach, and bell peppers. Non-starchy vegetables are low in calories and carbohydrates, making them an excellent choice for people with diabetes.

2.   Lean protein: Fill one-quarter of your plate with lean protein sources, such as chicken, fish, or tofu. Lean protein sources are low in saturated fat and can help keep you feeling full and satisfied.

3.   Starchy foods: Fill one-quarter of your plate with starchy foods, such as whole grains, potatoes, or rice. Limit your portion sizes of starchy foods, as they can cause a rapid increase in blood sugar levels.

Additional Tips for Balanced Eating

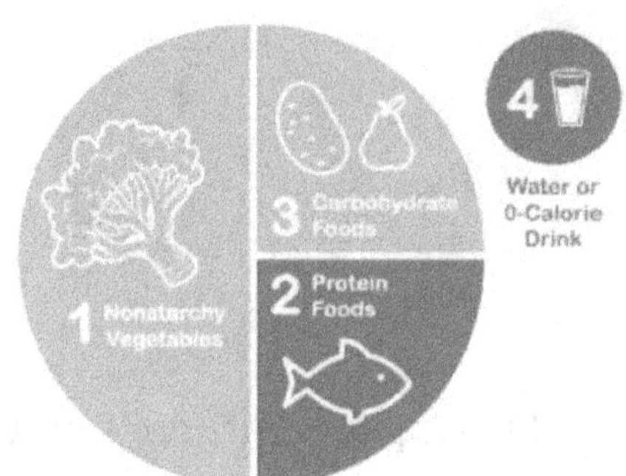

In addition to the Diabetes Plate Method, consider the following tips for balanced eating:

- Choose whole, unprocessed foods whenever possible.

- Limit your intake of added sugars and saturated fats.

- Incorporate healthy fats, such as avocados and nuts, into your diet.

- Drink plenty of water throughout the day.

- Consult with a registered dietitian or certified diabetes educator for personalized nutrition advice.

By following the Diabetes Plate Method and incorporating these additional tips, you can enjoy balanced, nutritious meals that support optimal blood sugar control.

About Portion Size

Portion size and serving sizes aren't always the same. A portion is the amount of food you choose to eat at one time, while a serving is a specific amount of food, such as one slice of bread or 8 ounces (1 cup) of milk.

These days, portions at restaurants are quite a bit larger than they were several years ago. One entrée can equal 3 or 4 servings! Studies show that people tend to eat more when they're served more food, so getting portions under control is really important for managing weight and blood sugar.

If you're eating out, have half of your meal wrapped up to go so you can enjoy it later. At home, measure out snacks; don't eat straight from the bag or box. At dinnertime, reduce the temptation to go back for seconds by keeping the serving bowls out of reach. And with this "handy" guide, you'll always have a way to estimate portion size at your fingertips:

1. **3 ounces of meat, fish, or poultry**
Palm of hand (no fingers)

2. **1 ounce of meat or cheese**
Thumb (tip to base)

3. **1 cup or 1 medium fruit**
Fist

4. **1–2 ounces of nuts or pretzels**
Cupped hand

5. **1 tablespoon** **Scan QR code for a**
Thumb tip (tip to 1st joint) **Downloadable meal**

6. **1** teaspoon **Planner**
Fingertip (tip to 1st joint)

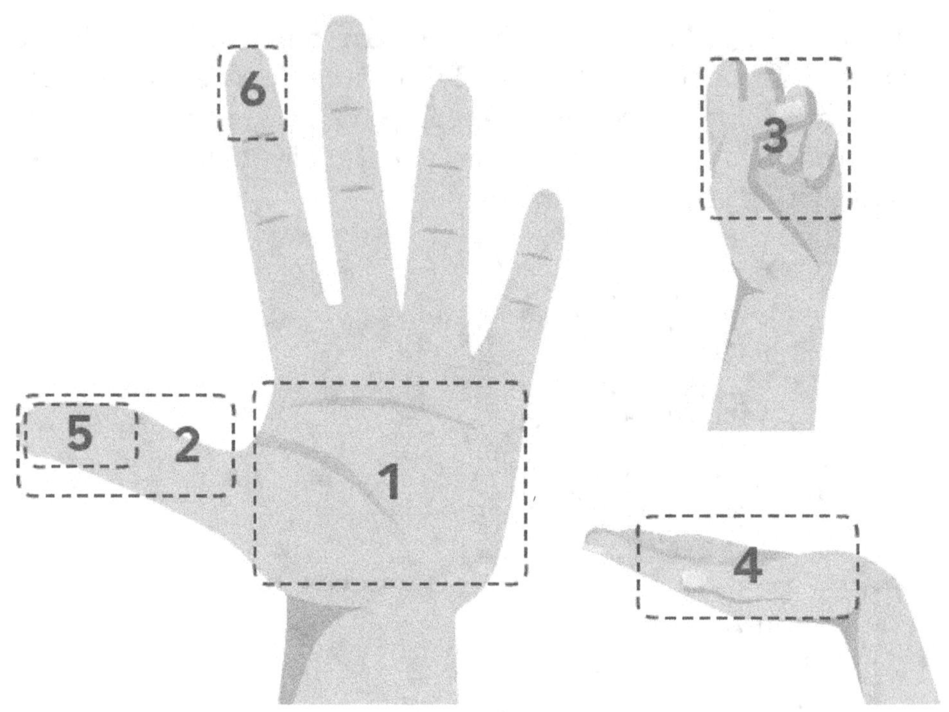

1. Understanding Carbohydrates: Carbohydrates are one of the main nutrients found in food and beverages. They are broken down into glucose (sugar) in the body, which is used as a primary source of energy. Carbohydrates are found in a wide variety of foods, including grains, fruits, vegetables, dairy products, and sweets.

2. Setting Carbohydrate Goals: The first step in carbohydrate counting is determining your carbohydrate goals, which are typically set in consultation with a healthcare professional such as a registered dietitian or certified diabetes educator. Your carbohydrate goals will depend on factors such as your

age, weight, activity level, medication regimen, and blood sugar targets.

3. Identifying Carbohydrate Sources: Carbohydrate counting involves identifying foods and beverages that contain carbohydrates and estimating the amount of carbohydrates in each serving. This includes foods like bread, pasta, rice, cereal, fruits, starchy vegetables, dairy products, sweets, and sugary beverages.

4. Portion Control: Once you've identified carbohydrate-containing foods, the next step is portion control. Portion sizes can vary depending on the food item, so it's important to measure or weigh foods to accurately determine serving sizes. Nutrition labels on packaged foods provide information on serving sizes and carbohydrate content per serving.

5. Counting Carbohydrates: Carbohydrates are typically measured in grams, and the total carbohydrate content of a food item is listed on its nutrition label. Carbohydrate counting involves keeping track of the total amount of carbohydrates consumed throughout the day and staying within your prescribed carbohydrate goals.

6. Monitoring Blood Sugar Levels: By tracking your carbohydrate intake and monitoring your blood sugar levels regularly, you can better understand how different foods affect your blood sugar and make adjustments to your diet as needed. It's im-

portant to work closely with your healthcare team to develop an individualized carbohydrate counting plan that meets your nutritional needs and helps you achieve your blood sugar targets.

Carbohydrate counting can be a flexible and effective way to manage blood sugar levels for individuals with diabetes, allowing for greater freedom and variety in food choices while still maintaining control over blood sugar levels.

Useful links.

1. MyFitnessPal - Offers a comprehensive database of foods with detailed nutritional information, including carbohydrate content. Users can track their daily food intake and set nutrition goals. Website: www.myfitnesspal.com

2. Calorie King - Provides nutritional information for thousands of foods, including carbohydrates, calories, and serving sizes. Users can search for specific foods or browse categories to plan meals. Website: www.calorieking.com

3. USDA Food Data Central - Offers a searchable database of nutrient information for thousands of foods, including carbohydrates. Users can search by food name, category, or nutrient content. Website: www.fdc.nal.usda.gov

4. Diabetes UK - Provides resources and tools for meal planning, including carbohydrate counting guides and recipe ideas. Website: www.diabetes.org.uk/guide-to-diabetes/enjoy-food

5. Eat This Much - Offers personalized meal plans

based on dietary preferences, calorie goals, and nutritional needs. Users can customize their meal plans to include specific amounts of carbohydrates. Website: www.eatthismuch.com

6. SparkPeople - Provides a variety of tools and resources for meal planning, including a food tracker and recipe database. Users can track their carbohydrate intake and monitor their overall nutrition. Website: www.sparkpeople.com

7. Atkins - Offers resources for low-carb meal planning, including recipes, meal plans, and educational articles. Website: www.atkins.com

8. Low Carb Program - Provides meal plans, recipes, and educational resources for people following a low-carbohydrate diet. Website: www.lowcarbprogram.com

9. Carb Manager - Offers a comprehensive tracking tool for monitoring carbohydrate intake, as well as recipes and meal planning features. Website: www.carbmanager.com

The Glycaemic Index Foundation - Provides information on the glycaemic index of foods and how it affects blood sugar levels. Users can search for foods by glycaemic index and plan meals accordingly. Website: www.gisymbol.com

Chapter 5

Exercise and Diabetes: Making Movement a Daily Habit

Regular exercise and physical activity are essential for effective diabetes management. Exercise can help improve insulin sensitivity, lower blood sugar levels, and reduce the risk of complications.

The Benefits of Exercise for People with Diabetes.

Exercise offers numerous benefits for people with diabetes, including:

- Improved insulin sensitivity: Regular exercise can help your body use insulin more efficiently, reducing the need for medication.

- Lower blood sugar levels: Exercise can help lower your blood sugar levels, both during and after physical activity.

- Weight management: Exercise can help you maintain a healthy weight or lose weight, reducing the risk of complications.

- Improved mood and mental health: Exercise can help reduce stress, anxiety, and depression, improving your overall quality of life.

Types of Exercise

There are various types of exercise that people with diabetes can enjoy, including:

- Aerobic exercise: Activities such as walking, jogging,

cycling, or swimming that increase your heart rate and breathing.

- Resistance training: Exercises that use weights, resistance bands, or your own body weight to build muscle.

- Flexibility exercises: Exercises that improve your range of motion and reduce stiffness, such as yoga or tai chi.

- Balance exercises: Exercises that improve your stability and reduce the risk of falls, such as balance training or heel-to-toe walking.

Tips for Exercising Safely with Diabetes

When exercising with diabetes, consider the following tips to stay safe and healthy:

- Check your blood sugar levels before and after exercise.

- Wear a medical ID bracelet or necklace that indicates you have diabetes.

- 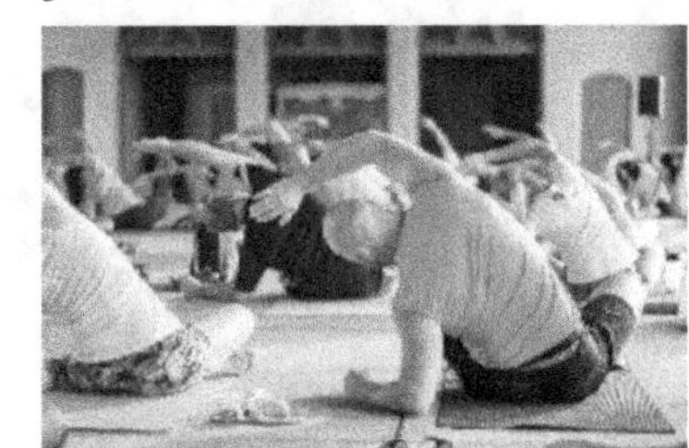

Carry a source of fast-acting carbohydrates, such as glucose tablets, in case of low blood sugar.

- Stay hydrated by drinking plenty of water.

- Warm up and cool down before and after exercise.

- Start slowly and gradually increase the intensity and duration of your workouts.

By making exercise a daily habit, you can enjoy numerous benefits for your physical and mental health. In the next chapter, we will explore medication management and the importance of taking your medications as prescribed. Also to plan balanced meals for optimal health.

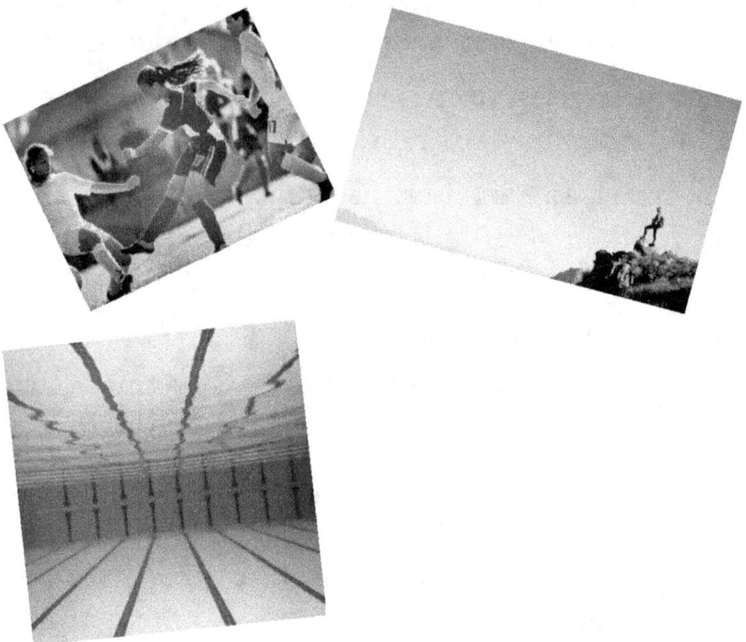

Chapter 6

Medication Management: Navigating Insulin and Other Medications

Taking medications as prescribed is a crucial aspect of effective diabetes management. Depending on your individual needs, your healthcare provider may prescribe insulin or other medications to help manage your blood sugar levels.

Insulin Therapy

Insulin therapy is a common treatment for people with Type 1 diabetes, as well as some people with Type 2 diabetes. There are various types of insulin available, including:

- Rapid-acting insulin: This type of insulin starts working within 15 minutes of injection and peaks after 1 hour.

- Short-acting insulin: This type of insulin starts working within 30 minutes of injection and peaks after 2 to 3 hours.

- Intermediate-acting insulin: This type of insulin starts working within 2 to 4 hours of injection and peaks after 4 to 12 hours.

- Long-acting insulin: This type of insulin starts working several hours after injection and provides steady insulin levels for up to 24 hours.

Your healthcare provider will determine the type and dose of insulin that is right for you based on your individual needs.

Other Medications for Diabetes

In addition to insulin, your healthcare provider may prescribe other medications to help manage your blood sugar levels, this is normally for type 2 diabetes. Some common medications include:

- Metformin: This medication helps reduce the amount of glucose produced by the liver and improves insulin sensitivity.

- Sulfonylureas: These medications stimulate the pancreas to produce more insulin.

- DPP-4 inhibitors: These medications help increase insulin production and reduce glucagon secretion.

- GLP-1 receptor agonists: These medications help slow down digestion, reduce appetite, and improve insulin sensitivity.

- SGLT2 inhibitors: These medications help the kidneys remove excess glucose from the body.

Tips for Medication Management

When managing medications for diabetes, consider the following tips:

- Take your medications as prescribed by your healthcare provider.

- Keep a record of your medications, including the name, dose, and frequency.

- Store your medications in a cool, dry place, away from direct sunlight.

- Check the expiration date of your medications and discard any that are past their expiration date.

- Consult with your healthcare provider before stopping or changing any medications.

By following these tips for medication management, you can help ensure that your medications are working effectively to manage your blood sugar levels. In the next chapter, we will explore strategies for managing mental health and emotional well-being with diabetes.

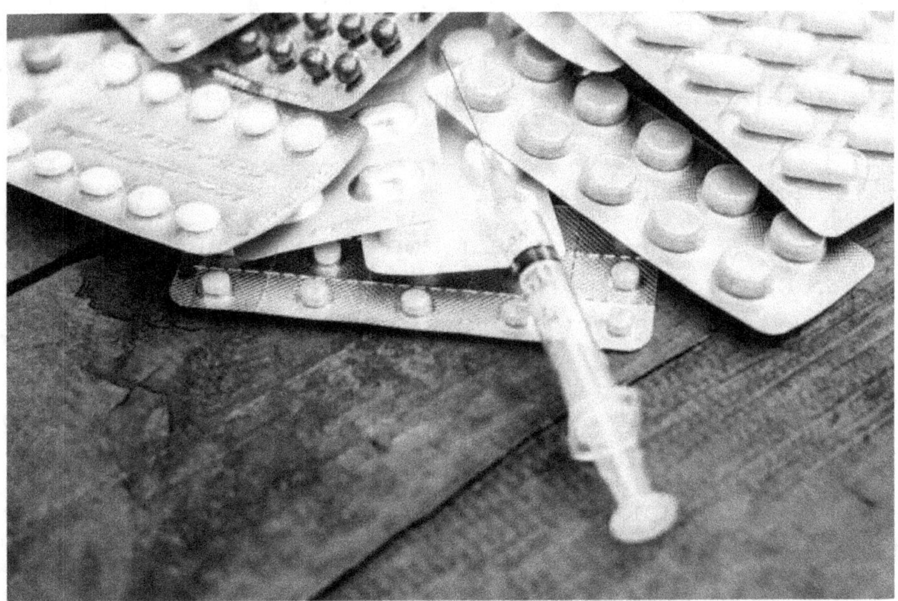

<h1 style="text-align:center">Chapter 7</h1>

Mental Health and Diabetes: Strategies for Emotional Well-being

Living with diabetes can be challenging, both physically and emotionally. In this chapter, we will explore strategies for managing mental health and emotional well-being with diabetes.

The Emotional Impact of Diabetes

Diabetes can have a significant emotional impact, causing feelings of stress, anxiety, and depression. These feelings can make it more challenging to manage your condition effectively, leading to poor blood sugar control and an increased risk of complications.

Coping Strategies for Diabetes

To cope with the emotional challenges of living with diabetes, consider the following strategies:

- Practice mindfulness meditation or deep breathing exercises to reduce stress and anxiety.

- Join a support group for people with diabetes to connect with others who understand your experiences.

- Engage in regular physical activity to improve your mood and mental health.

- Practice self-care, such as getting enough sleep, eating a healthy diet, and taking time for relaxation and enjoyment.

- Consult with a mental health professional, such as a

therapist or counsellor, for additional support and guidance.

Tips for Communicating with Your Healthcare Provider

Effective communication with your healthcare provider is essential for managing your mental health and emotional well-being with diabetes. Consider the following tips:

- Be honest and open about your feelings and concerns.
- Ask questions and seek clarification about your condition and treatment options.
- Bring a list of your medications and any symptoms you are experiencing.
- Discuss any lifestyle factors that may be impacting your mental health, such as stress, sleep, or diet.
- Work with your healthcare provider to develop a personalized care plan that addresses both your physical and emotional health.

By following these strategies and tips, you can manage the emotional challenges of living with diabetes and improve your overall quality of life. In the next chapter, we will explore the importance of building a support system and seeking help when needed.

Chapter 8

Building a Support System: Friends, Family, and Healthcare Professionals

Managing diabetes can be challenging, and having a strong support system in place is essential for your success. In this chapter, we will explore the importance of building a support system and seeking help when needed.

The Role of Friends and Family

Friends and family can play a critical role in your diabetes management. They can provide emotional support, encouragement, and practical help, such as reminding you to take your medications or preparing healthy meals.

To build a strong support system with your friends and family, consider the following tips:

- Communicate openly and honestly about your needs and concerns.

- Educate your loved ones about diabetes and how it affects your life.

- Encourage your loved ones to attend doctor's appointments and support groups with you.

- Share your successes and challenges with your loved ones, and seek their feedback and advice.

The Role of Healthcare Professionals

Healthcare professionals, such as doctors, nurses, and dietitians, can provide expert guidance and support for your diabetes management. They can help you develop a personalized care plan, monitor your condition, and adjust your treatment as needed.
To build a strong support system with your healthcare professionals, consider the following tips:

- Choose healthcare professionals who are knowledgeable and experienced in diabetes care.
- Communicate openly and honestly with your healthcare professionals about your condition and treatment options.
- Follow your healthcare professionals' advice and recommendations, and ask questions if you are unsure or have concerns.
- Keep a record of your appointments, medications, and test results to share with your healthcare professionals.

Seeking Help When Needed

Asking for help is not a sign of weakness, but rather a strength. If you are struggling to manage your diabetes or experiencing emotional challenges, don't hesitate to seek help.
Consider reaching out to:

- Your healthcare provider for medical advice and support.
- A mental health professional, such as a therapist or counsellor, for additional support and guidance.
- A support group for people with diabetes to connect with others who understand your experiences.

By building a strong support system and seeking help when needed, you can improve your diabetes management and enhance your overall quality of life. In the next chapter, we will explore healthy habits for life and tips for long-term success.

Chapter 9

Healthy Habits for Life: Tips for Long-term Success

Effective diabetes management requires ongoing effort and commitment. In this chapter, we will explore healthy habits for life and tips for long-term success.

Eat a Healthy Diet

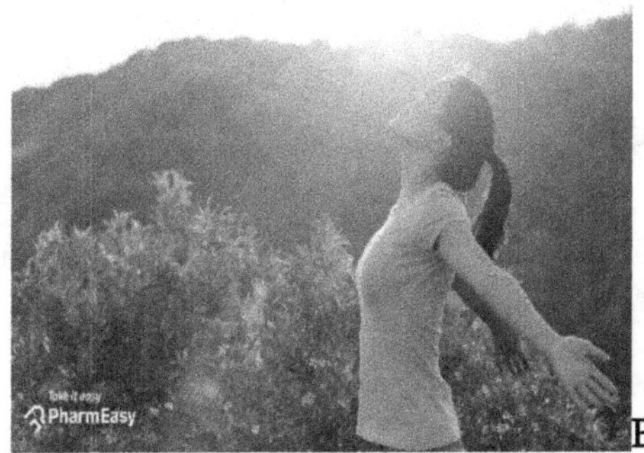

Eating a healthy, balanced diet is essential for managing your blood sugar levels and preventing complications. A healthy diet should include:

- Plenty of vegetables, fruits, and whole grains
- Lean protein sources, such as chicken, fish, and tofu
- Healthy fats, such as avocado, nuts, and olive oil
- Limited processed and high-sugar foods

Engage in Regular Physical Activity

Regular physical activity can help improve your insulin sensitivity, reduce your blood sugar levels, and prevent complications.

Aim for at least 30 minutes of moderate-intensity exercise, such as brisk walking, most days of the week.

Monitor Your Blood Sugar Levels

Monitoring your blood sugar levels is essential for managing your condition and preventing complications. Work with your health-care provider to develop a personalized testing schedule and goals.

Get Enough Sleep

Getting enough sleep is essential for your overall health and well-being. Aim for 7-8 hours of sleep each night, and establish a consistent sleep routine.

Manage Stress

Managing stress is essential for your emotional and physical health. Consider practicing mindfulness meditation, yoga, or other relaxation techniques to reduce stress and improve your overall well-being.

Stay Motivated

Staying motivated can be challenging, but it is essential for long-term success. Consider setting small, achievable goals, tracking your progress, and celebrating your successes.

Stay Informed

Follow a low-carb eating plan	Try out this <u>superfood</u> for energy and health	Track your progress to stay motivated
Always check food labels for sugar and carbs	Replace your morning coffee and milk with cinnamon tea	Eat slowly, without any interference
Try to exercise at least 3 times a week	Detox 2 to 4 times a year.	Drink more water to increase your weight loss
Have a high protein breakfast	Include superfoods to at least one meal a day	Believe in yourself

Staying informed about the latest research, treatments, and technologies can help you manage your condition more effectively. Consider attending support groups, webinars, or conferences, and following trusted diabetes websites and organizations.

By following these healthy habits for life and tips for long-term success, you can manage your diabetes effectively and enhance your overall quality of life. Remember, effective diabetes management is a journey, not a destination. Stay committed, stay motivated, and seek support when needed.

Chapter 10

Embracing Your Diabetes Journey: A Path to Optimal Health

Living with diabetes can be challenging, but it is also an opportunity for growth, learning, and self-discovery. By understanding your condition, developing a personalized care plan, and building a strong support system, you can take control of your health and embrace your diabetes journey.

Throughout this eBook, we have explored various aspects of diabetes self-care, from monitoring your blood sugar levels to building a support system and cultivating healthy habits for the long term. By following the tips and strategies outlined in this eBook, you can:

- Understand your condition and its impact on your health
- Develop a personalized care plan that meets your individual needs
- Build a strong support system of friends, family, and healthcare professionals
- Practice healthy habits for life, such as eating a healthy diet, engaging in regular physical activity, and managing stress
- Stay motivated and committed to your long-term success
- Stay informed about the latest research, treatments, and technologies

Remember, managing diabetes is a journey, not a destination. Stay committed, stay motivated, and seek support when needed. With the right tools, knowledge, and support, you can live a vibrant, fulfilling life with diabetes.

Thank you for reading this eBook. We hope that it has provided you with valuable insights, strategies, and inspiration for your diabetes journey.

Useful links

1. American Diabetes Association (ADA) - United States - Provides information on diabetes management, research updates, advocacy efforts, and community support. Website: www.diabetes.org

2. Diabetes UK - United Kingdom - Offers resources on diabetes prevention, management, and support services. Website: www.diabetes.org.uk

3. International Diabetes Federation (IDF) - Global - Provides global diabetes statistics, advocacy initiatives, and educational resources for healthcare professionals and people living with diabetes. Website: www.idf.org

4. National Institute of Diabetes and Digestive and Kidney Diseases (NIDDK) - United States - Offers comprehensive information on diabetes research, prevention, and treatment options. Website: www.niddk.nih.gov

5. Diabetes Canada - Canada - Provides information on diabetes management, support programs, and advocacy efforts. Website: www.diabetes.ca

6. Diabetes Australia - Australia - Offers resources

on diabetes management, prevention, and support services. Website: www.diabetesaustralia.com.au

7. European Association for the Study of Diabetes (EASD) - Europe - Provides diabetes research updates, guidelines, and educational resources for healthcare professionals and researchers. Website: www.easd.org

8. Juvenile Diabetes Research Foundation (JDRF) - Global - Focuses on funding research to find a cure for type 1 diabetes and provides support for people living with the condition. Website: www.jdrf.org

9. Mayo Clinic - United States - Offers comprehensive information on diabetes diagnosis, treatment options, and lifestyle management tips. Website: www.mayoclinic.org/diseases-conditions/diabetes

10. Diabetes.co.uk - United Kingdom - Provides information on diabetes management, forums for peer support, and resources for healthcare professionals. Website: www.diabetes.co.uk

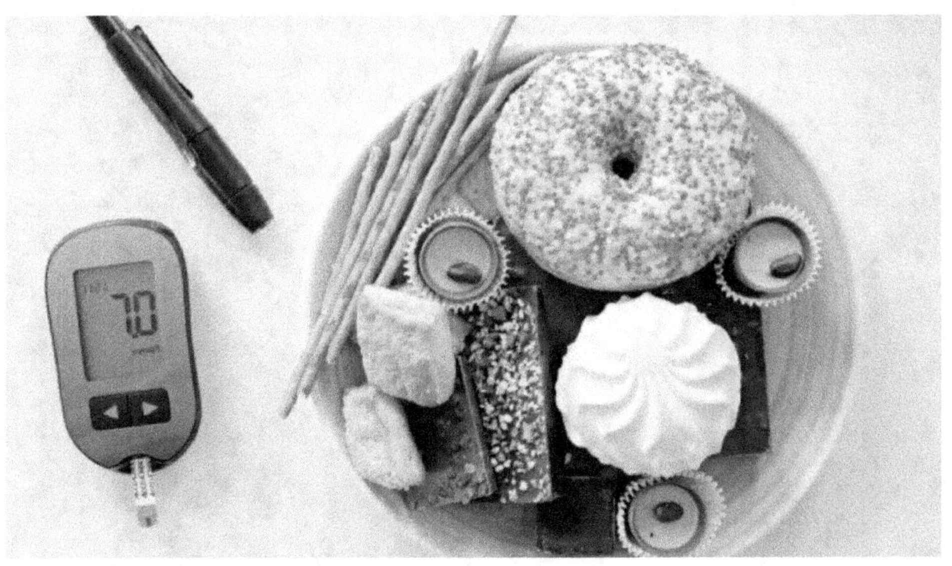